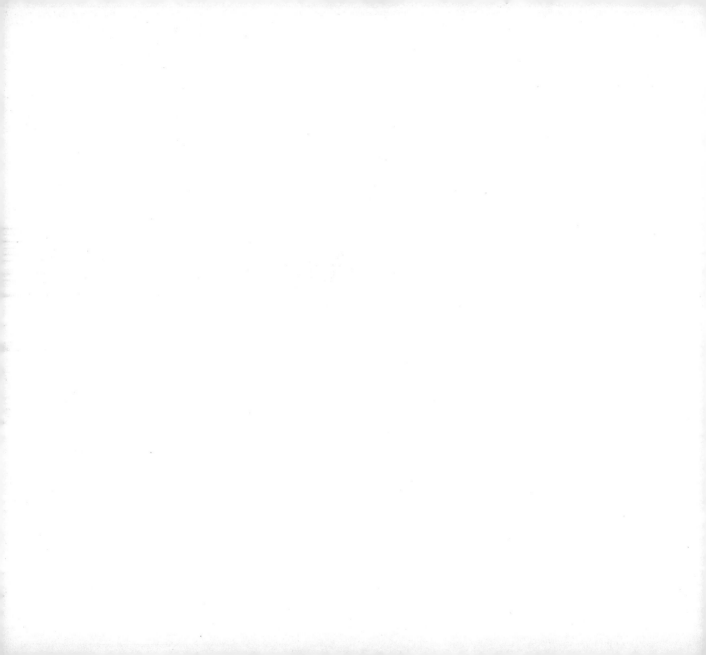

Our Bodies

Our Muscles

Charlotte Guillain

Heinemann Library
Chicago, Illinois

www.heinemannraintree.com
Visit our website to find out
more information about
Heinemann-Raintree books.

To order:

☎ Phone 888-454-2279

💻 Visit www.heinemannraintree.com
   to browse our catalog and order online.

Editorial: Rebecca Rissman, Laura Knowles, Nancy Dickmann,
  and Sian Smith
Picture research: Ruth Blair and Mica Brancic
Designed by Joanna Hinton-Malivoire
Original Illustrations © Capstone Global Library Ltd. 2010
Illustrated by Tony Wilson
Printed and bound by Leo Paper Group

14 13 12 11 10
10 9 8 7 6 5 4 3 2 1

Library of Congress Cataloging-in-Publication Data
Guillain, Charlotte.
  Our muscles / Charlotte Guillain.
     p. cm. -- (Our bodies)
  Includes bibliographical references and index.
  ISBN 978-1-4329-3593-1 (hc) -- ISBN 978-1-4329-3602-0 (pb)
1. Muscles--Juvenile literature. I. Title.
  QP321.G92 2010
  612.7'4--dc22
                       2009022297

Acknowledgments
The author and publisher are grateful to the following for
permission to reproduce copyright material:
© Capstone Global Library p.**8** (Karon Dubke); Corbis pp.**11** (©
David Stoecklein), **20** (© Lisa B.), **22** (© John Lund/Sam Diephuis/
Blend Images); iStockphoto pp.**10**, **9** (© Alexander Yakovlev), **17** (©
Rosemarie Gearhart); Photolibrary pp.**5** (© HillCreek Pictures BV), **15**
(© Rafael Guerrero/Index Stock Imagery), **16** (© OJO Images), **21** (©
Banana Stock); Science Photo Library p.**14** (© David Constantine);
Shutterstock pp.**13** (© Mandy Godbehear), **18** (© Ostanina Ekaterina
Vadimovna).

Front cover photograph of children with hoops reproduced with
permission of Corbis (© Randy Faris). Back cover photograph
reproduced with permission of iStockphoto.

Every effort has been made to contact copyright holders of any
material reproduced in this book. Any omissions will be rectified in
subsequent printings if notice is given to the publisher.

Contents

Body Parts

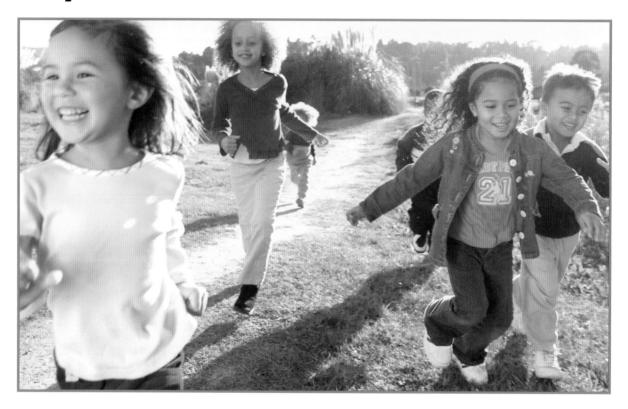

Our bodies have many parts.

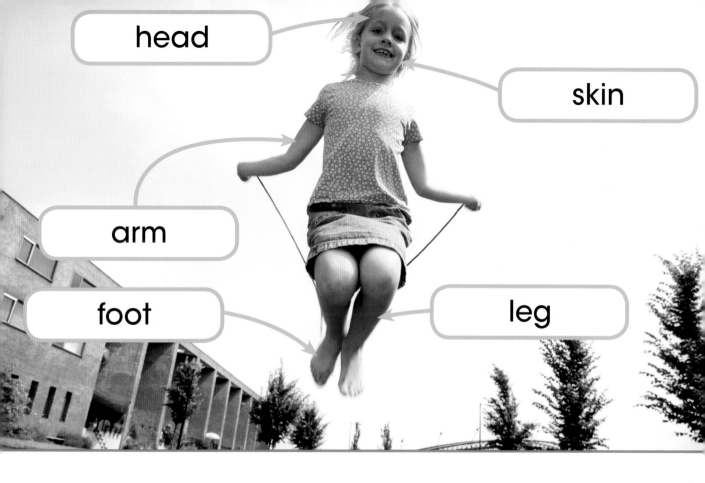

head

skin

arm

foot

leg

Our bodies have parts on
the outside.

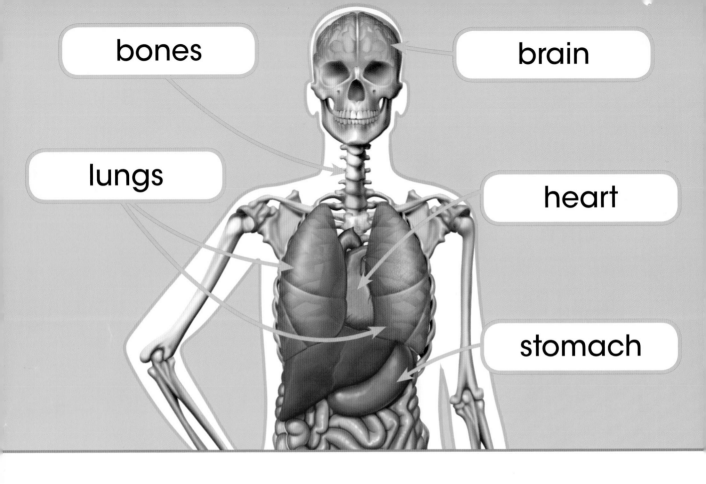

bones

brain

lungs

heart

stomach

Our bodies have parts on the inside.

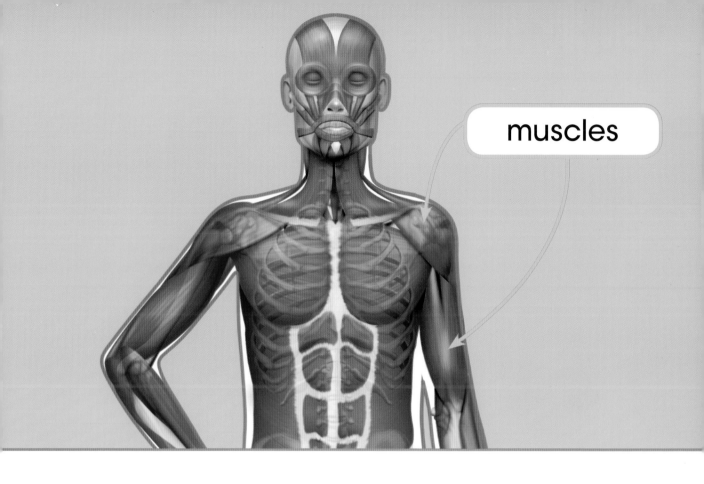

muscles

Your muscles are inside your body.

Your Muscles

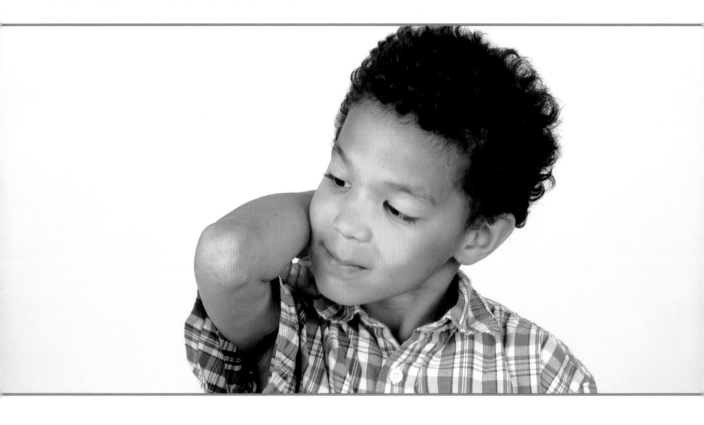

You cannot see most of
your muscles.

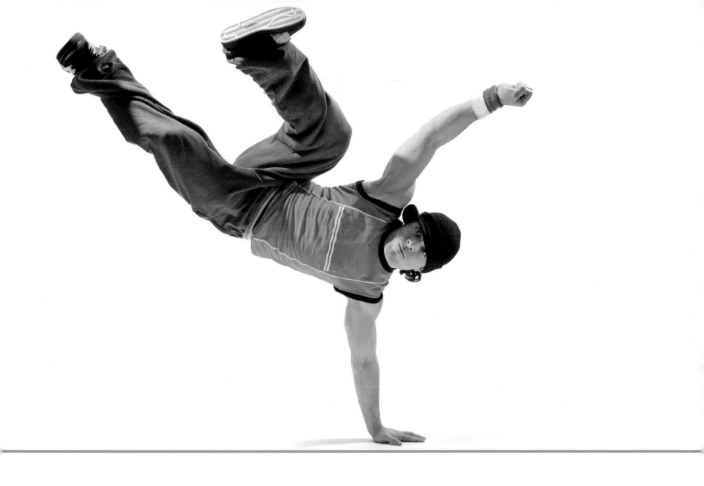

Your muscles are all over your body.

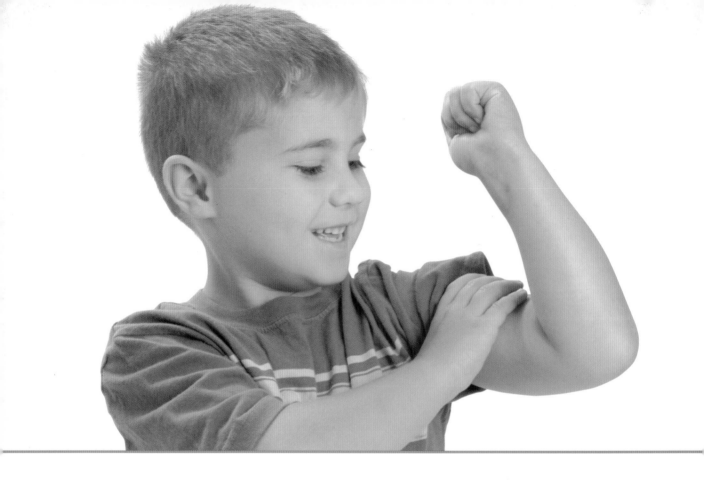

You can feel your muscles.

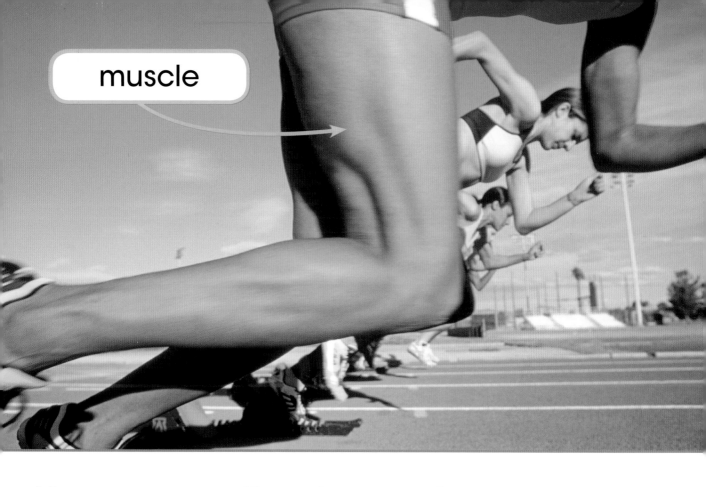

muscle

You can see the shape of some muscles.

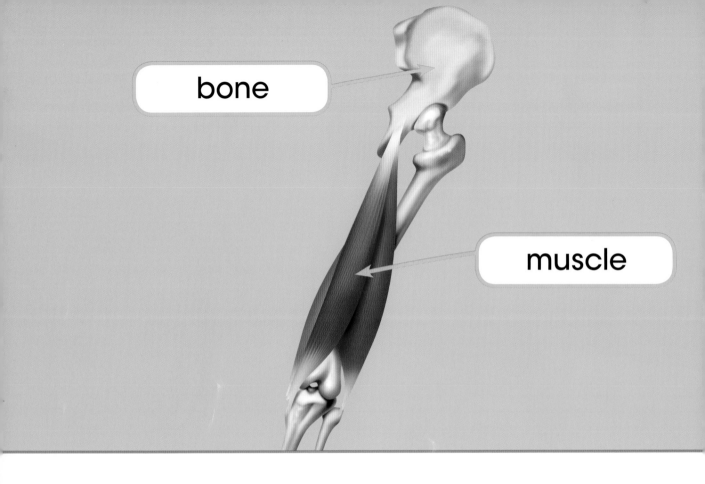

bone

muscle

Some muscles are joined to your bones.

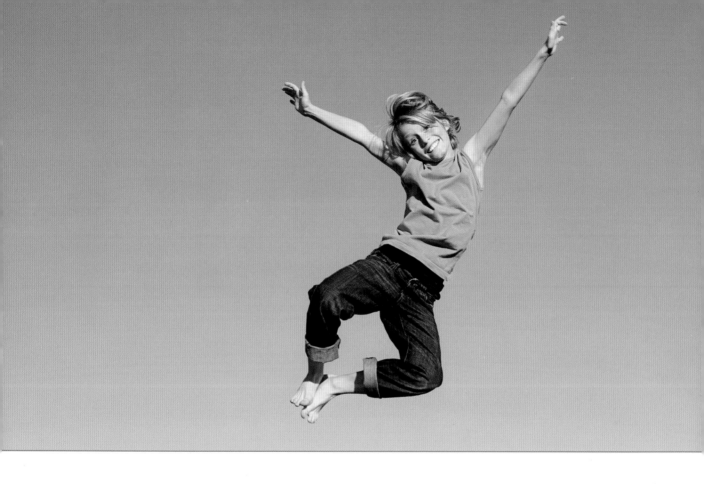

The muscles pull on your bones to make them move.

What Do Muscles Do?

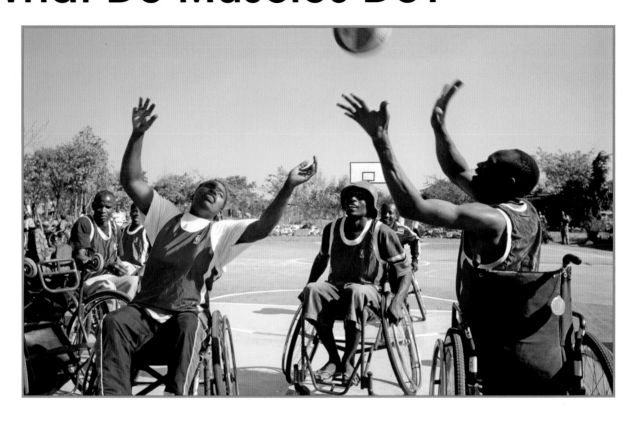

Your muscles make your
body move.

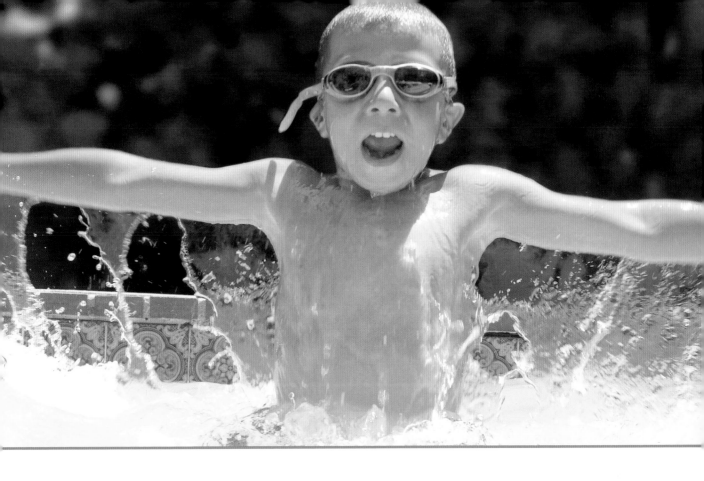

You can choose to move
some muscles.

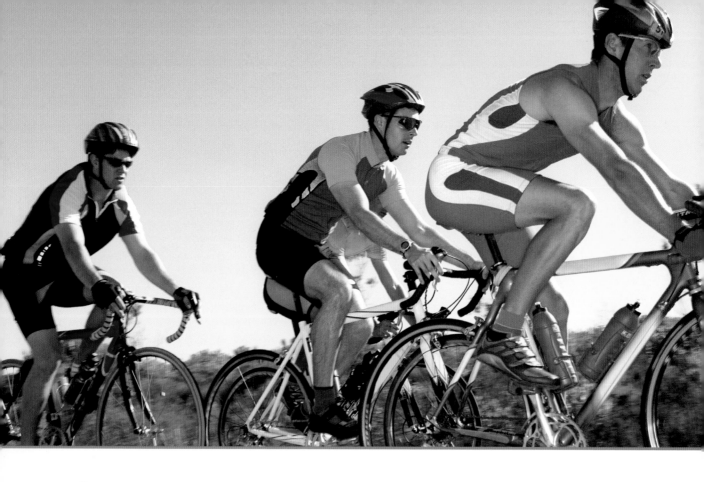

Some muscles help you
move around.

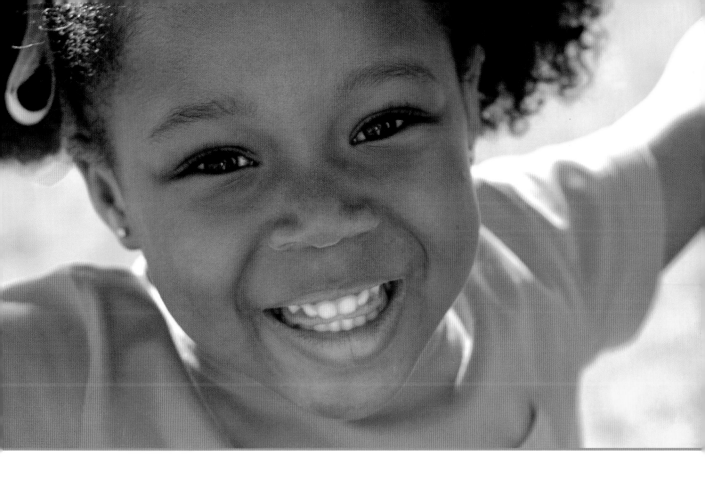

Some muscles help you smile.

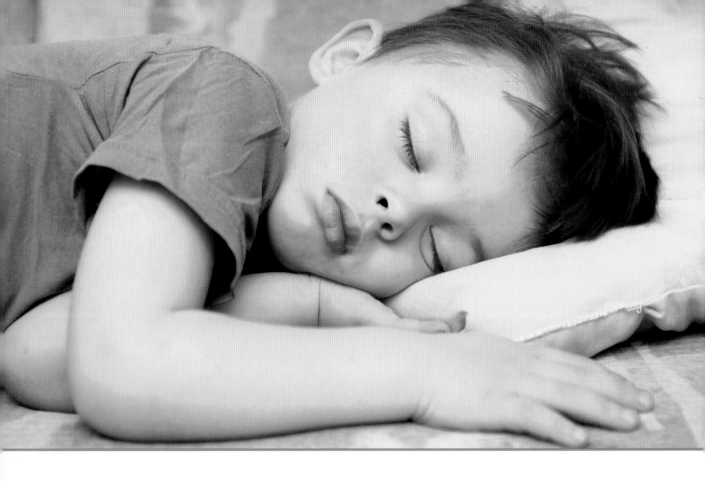

Some muscles work all the time.

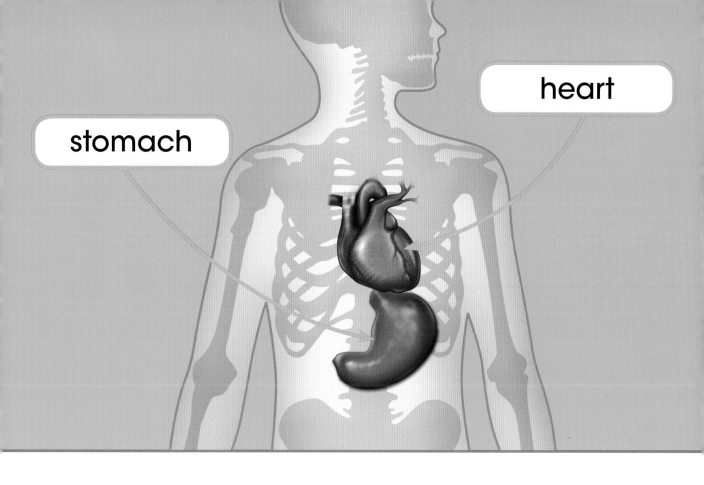

stomach

heart

Your heart and stomach muscles
work all the time.

Staying Healthy

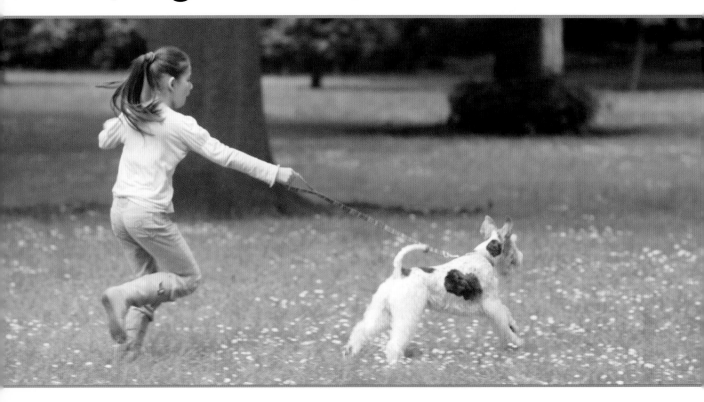

You can exercise to help
your muscles.

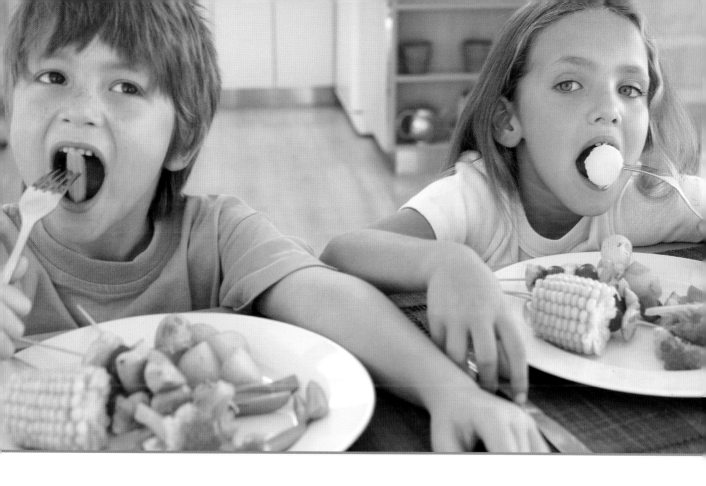

You can eat healthy food to help your muscles.

Quiz

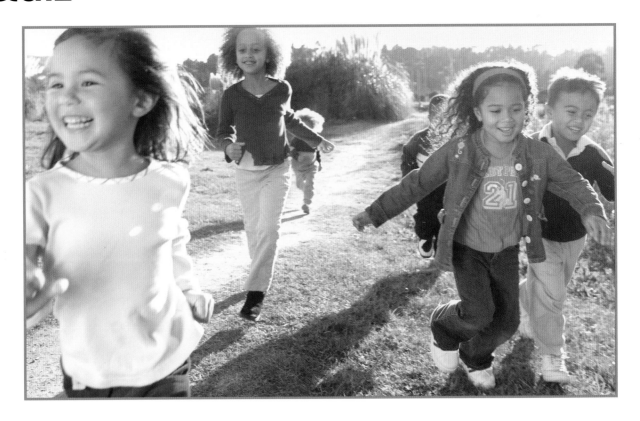

Where in your body are
your muscles?

Answer on page 24

Picture Glossary

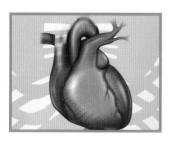 **heart** a muscle inside your chest. Your heart beats all the time so that it can push blood around your body.

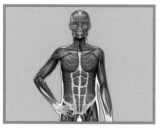 **muscles** stretchy parts inside your body. Some muscles help you to move your body.

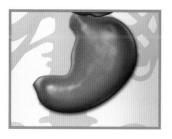 **stomach** a muscle inside your body. Your stomach breaks food into tiny bits so that your body can use it.

Index

Answer to quiz on page 22:
Your muscles are inside your body.

Notes to parents and teachers

Before reading

Ask children to name the parts of their body they can see on the outside. Then ask them what parts of their body are inside. Make a list of them together and see if the children know what each body part does, for example, stomachs break down food. Discuss where their muscles are and see if anyone knows what muscles are for.

After reading

- Ask the children to step up and down or do jumping jacks for a minute (timed by you). When they have stopped, ask how their legs feel. Discuss how exercise can make our muscles ache and the importance of not straining our muscles.
- Put the children into pairs and ask them to count how many times the other child blinks in a minute (timed by you). Compare the answers and then explain how a muscle in our eyes makes us blink without thinking. Discuss why we need this muscle to work like this.